# The Breastfeeding Diaries

Edited by
## Kate Davis
"The Funny Mommy"

 Meadowbrook Press
Distributed by Simon & Schuster
New York

Library of Congress Cataloging-in-Publication Data

The breastfeeding diaries : real moms share their funniest misadventures /
edited by Kate Davis.
  p. cm.
  Summary: "Real moms–and even a dad–share their funny-but-true
misadventures involving breastfeeding"–Provided by publisher.
  ISBN-10 0-88166-508-8, ISBN-13 978-0-88166-508-6 (Meadowbrook Press)
  ISBN-10 0-684-04364-5, ISBN-13 978-0-684-04364-7 (Simon & Schuster)
  1. Breastfeeding–Humor.  I. Davis, Kate, 1967-
RJ216.B7783 2007
649'.33–dc22

                              2007029078

Coordinating Editors: Christine Zuchora-Walske, Angela Wiechmann
Copyeditor: Alicia Ester
Proofreader: Megan McGinnis
Production Manager: Paul Woods
Graphic Design Manager: Tamara Peterson
Cover and Interior Illustrations: B. K. Taylor

© 2007 by Meadowbrook Creations

Published by Meadowbrook Press, 5451 Smetana Drive, Minnetonka, Minnesota 55343

www.meadowbrookpress.com

BOOK TRADE DISTRIBUTION by Simon and Schuster, a division of Simon
and Schuster, Inc., 1230 Avenue of the Americas, New York, New York 10020

10 09 08 07   10 9 8 7 6 5 4 3 2 1

Printed in the United States of America

To breastfeeding moms
everywhere—never
forget to laugh

# Acknowledgments

We'd like to thank the following
nursing mothers who reviewed
stories for this anthology:

Stephanie Ray Brown
Jane Davidson
Joanne Hartman
Jeanine Ketch
Mary Krebsturnbull
Signe Lansky
Darlene Mueller
Michelle Owens
Tami Peterson
Stacie Ralston
Jana O'Leary Sullivan
Annamarie K. Tabery
Danielle White
Faye Whyte

# Contents

# Introduction

I'm a standup comedian and, more importantly, a mother of three. When you add it up, I've spent three years of my life being pregnant and postpartum, four years breastfeeding, ten years trying to lose the weight, and twelve years wondering what happened to my Tupperware lids. I think the show *Survivor* shouldn't take place on an island, but in a new nursing mom's home.

As I screened the true-to-life anecdotes in this anthology, I couldn't help but remember the hilarious breastfeeding moments I myself have experienced—like the time I was back doing standup nine weeks after giving birth to my beautiful (you always have to throw in that adjective, even if your baby is ugly) baby girl. I was doing a comedy show out of town, and I had prepared the best I could. By that I mean I had put on a good bra and nursing pads—when I let down, I was like a Guinness tap in an Irish pub on Saint Paddy's Day.

I was working that night with a very talented young comic named Jason Rouse. He's tattooed, pierced, and, more times than not, naked by the end of his show. If you've ever seen the movie or TV show *Jackass*, he's a lot like those guys. He's known for peeing in a water bottle, and if he *really* wants to shock you, he'll drink it—or so the rumor goes. As my cue music began, I turned to wish Jason luck with his show, but suddenly his jaw dropped and his face went flush. He pointed to my shirt, staring in horror yet trying to avert his eyes at the same time. My light-gray shirt now had black circles around my breasts, and milk was streaming out with a good five-foot range.

I pressed my elbows to my breasts and looked at him with disbelief: The man who embraced every bodily function had been taken down by a mom and her breast milk. I laughed, telling him if the audience didn't like me, I'd shoot them with my "breast guns," and that I'd be *milking* my jokes all night. Of course, I wasn't worried. I'm a mom—I had brought a black sweater, which I quickly threw on as I walked on the stage.

From comedy stages to the many stages of mother-hood, reading these hilarious tales will bring back embarrassing-yet-funny memories for any veteran nursing mom. If you're a mom-to-be eagerly awaiting your first nursing experience, then these funnier-than-fiction stories will give you a glimpse of what to expect.

You'll read about leaking, squirting, flashing, and other common breastfeeding mishaps. Wait till you find out how one mom earned the nickname "Squirts" and what happened to a pumping mom who forgot her business meeting was by videoconference. You'll also read about sleep-deprived nights, such as the time a zombie-like mom thought she was carrying her baby, when really she was cradling her breast down the hall. Now *that's* tired! There are laugh-out-loud tales about nursing in public—did you know breastfeeding could get you out of a parking ticket? You'll also learn how breastfeeding affects people around you, including dads, kids, relatives, coworkers, and perfect strangers. In fact, one group of moms and their nursing babies suddenly became an "exhibit" at an art museum.

Some women—especially first-time nursing moms— might think these misadventures are mortifying, horrifying, and impossible to live down. But as you read this book, I hope you understand the stories aren't *tragedies*—they're *comedies*. These stories cracked me up and also touched me because I, as well, have been that exhausted, that flustered, that engorged. I, too, have been caught with a breast hanging out.

So every time you squirt someone across the room, leak through your shirt during a meeting, or show a waiter more than he or you bargained for, remember to laugh out loud. Me, I've made a career of making fun of my mothering mishaps. And remember, you're not the first nursing mom to experience these moments, and you won't be the last. Enjoy your big, milky breasts and your voluptuous body. Treasure every moment—the good, the bad, and the leaky.

—Kate Davis,
"The Funny Mommy"

PS: Speaking of "leaky," let's start the fun with a story about the time I turned a hot tub into a "shower" at my local gym. Enjoy!

# The Workout

I gained eighty pounds during my pregnancy. I know—I should have given birth to an eight-year-old. After my merely six-pound, fourteen-ounce baby was born, I was determined to lose the weight.

I had girlfriends who could fit back into their pre-pregnancy jeans two weeks after giving birth, exclaiming, "I weigh less now than I did before I had the baby!" Meanwhile, I wore extendable-stomach pants and tried to avoid making eye contact when people asked me when I was due...while I pushed my newborn in her stroller.

So my extendable-stomach pants and I made our way to the local gym. I was hooked up with a snotty trainer named Amber who looked no older than nineteen and no larger than a size zero.

She started me on the treadmill. It began slowly, and I thought to myself, "I can do this." That confidence lasted all of ten seconds. The machine suddenly sped up, and the faster it went, the faster my size-H boobs (that's right, size H) flew, almost giving me a black eye with each stride. Amber had walked off, and I was stuck.

Not being familiar with the treadmill, I nervously pulled the emergency ripcord. (I was terrified of what was going to happen: Would an alarm go off? Would I catapult over the treadmill to land on the hot trainer across the gym?) As the treadmill came to a jolting stop, I decided to make a run for the locker room. I quickly whipped off my workout gear and covered myself with a towel, hoping Amber wouldn't come looking for me.

There was a hot tub in the locker room, and that excited me more than anything. I decided to have a soak, followed by a long shower, during which I'd shave my legs without interruption (a luxury in my world at that time). The hot tub was pretty crowded with about six women winding down in it. For some reason, the club didn't allow bathing suits, so I stripped, made my way in, and sank down in ecstasy. Amber would never find me here.

After a couple of minutes of bliss, I heard a shriek. I opened my eyes to see a woman pointing at me—and my breast milk hitting her right below her lip.

"You're leaking! You're spraying from your breasts!" she screamed as she leapt out of the hot tub. The others followed quickly, screaming similar things, while I continued spraying like Niagara Falls.

I wasn't scheduled to nurse for an hour, but I guess the heat had affected my breasts. I timidly made my way out, holding my breasts while my milk dripped to the ground from between my fingers. What flew out of my mouth next shocked me: "It's okay, really. I don't think there are *that* many calories in breast milk, and it's a great facial cleaner."

As I grabbed my towel, I looked up to see the club manager and Amber standing there with my breast milk victims behind them. I felt as if I were in the Old West, about to be run out of town. And I was. The manager politely asked me to leave and refunded my membership fees as they drained the hot tub. I left with my extendable-stomach pants and the fond memory of "I don't think there are *that* many calories in breast milk...."

I eventually lost the weight through Rollerblading and walking with a sports stroller. I have yet to enter another hot tub.

—Kate Davis, "The Funny Mommy"

# Conference Call

⬤ ⬤ ⬤ ⬤ ⬤ ⬤ ⬤ ⬤ ⬤ ⬤ ⬤ ⬤ ⬤ ⬤ ⬤ ⬤ ⬤ ⬤ ⬤ ⬤ ⬤ ⬤ ⬤ ⬤

I have a private office at work, so I've never had to worry about finding a place to pump discreetly. Occasionally, I must attend conference calls in a separate conference room, but that's private as well—or so I thought.

Last week, I had a scheduled call with our parent company's board of directors. I entered the conference room, set up my pump, and prepared myself for pumping. (I like to put up my feet and close my eyes.) As I began to pump, I heard the call starting. There was dead silence after I said "hello," so I opened my eyes and turned bright red.

It was a *video*conference, not a telephone conference. There were eight people on the television screen, averting their eyes. I started laughing, so they did, too. I turned the video camera toward the wall until I finished pumping, then proceeded with the call.

Though it was embarrassing initially, I think it loosened everyone up. Still, I think I'll pump with my eyes open from now on.

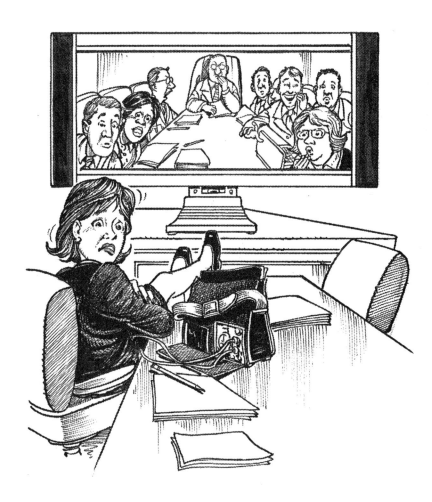

# What's for Lunch?

I was baby-sitting my niece Lauren, an energetic four-year-old. She was very excited about her new cousin, Breanna. Lauren asked about everything I did with Breanna, following me around excitedly, much to the chagrin of my three-year-old, Autumn, who desperately wanted to play with her older cousin.

Around 11:30, the girls asked when we were going to have lunch. I explained that I needed to feed the baby her lunch first. Lauren went to the kitchen, eagerly waiting for me to pull out baby food. When I went to the couch with Breanna and set her on my lap, Lauren looked confused.

"What are you doing?" she asked.

"Giving Breanna her lunch."

Although I tried to be discreet about it, Lauren could see Breanna's lunch was not coming from the refrigerator.

"What are you *doing*?" Lauren looked mortified.

"I'm giving her milk. This is her lunch."

Lauren seemed to lose interest and ran off to play with Autumn, who was quite used to seeing me nurse Breanna.

After about fifteen minutes, I prepared a couple grilled cheese sandwiches and some fruit and called the girls to lunch. Autumn came quickly, but Lauren didn't.

After waiting a few minutes, I called to Lauren again but she didn't come. Eventually I went and found her quietly playing. She didn't look at me. "Lauren, aren't you coming to have lunch?"

"No."

"Honey, it's all ready. Come on."

"No."

"You just told me you were hungry, Lauren. I have everything ready."

She looked at me very strangely. "Do we eat on the couch?"

"We could eat in the living room if you want to," I said.

Suddenly she burst into tears. "I don't want milk!" she cried.

Then I got it. Lauren thought her lunch was going to be breast milk as well!

# Grace

M y two-year-old son, Michael, has always been a precocious talker. He speaks in very clear, complete sentences and learns something new every day. We have enjoyed natural weaning, and he has methodically dropped feedings on his own as he has grown.

We always say a blessing at dinnertime when all three of us are home. Michael has been learning to hold our hands and say a simple blessing followed by "amen."

Several mornings ago, I got him out of his crib and brought him into our bedroom. He asked to eat, and as I prepared to nurse him, he spontaneously said, "Thank you, God, for the food. Amen!"

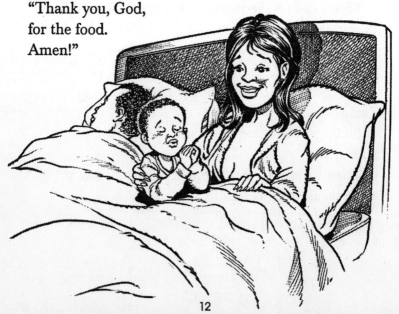

# Got Cream?

After my first child was born, my breasts produced so much milk that I was constantly leaking and the skin around my nipples was painfully cracked. The only way to help soothe my skin was to go without a top. When company came over, I would wear something, but with my mom or sisters, I would just drape a towel over myself.

One day, my mother and I were having coffee and my towel fell. In an attempt to grab the towel, I accidentally applied pressure to one of my breasts. Milk shot across the table.

My mother dryly said, "No, thanks. You know I take my coffee black."

# The Buzz and the Boss

I returned to work when my daughter was three months old, and I used a breast pump to express milk several times a day. My first day back was actually my first day as the new boss. That meant I had the privilege of a private office—with floor-to-ceiling windows that luckily had blinds.

I didn't really know the people who worked in the cubicles and workspaces outside my office window, and they certainly didn't know me. They knew I had a young baby, but they didn't quite understand what that might mean. This was especially true for the employee whose desk was directly outside my office. He seemed curious when he saw me fiddling with the ancient set of Venetian blinds atop my office windows, but looked relieved when I lowered them.

At the appointed hour, I hung a sign on my office door, saying I'd be out in about fifteen minutes, and closed my door. Sitting comfortably with the day's newspaper spread out on the desk in front of me, I began my pumping ritual: open shirt and bra, apply undignified pump parts to breasts, switch machine on, wait. The pump, which had already seen a full year of service when my now-three-year-old son was a baby, was a bit noisier than before. In fact, it rhythmically hummed and whirred and buzzed on my wooden desk until I had filled two bottles of milk. I then stored the milk, rearranged my bra and shirt, and opened my office door. The employee stationed near my door happened to be glancing up, and I gave him a big, perhaps somewhat sheepish, smile.

The next few times, all went well. I figured the noise didn't matter, as I had the thick glass windows between me and everyone else. And when I was sequestered in my office, nobody seemed to miss me (though they did tend to line up outside with questions, waiting for me to come out).

One of those times, I opened my office door to see a few men gathered around my neighboring employee's desk, nudging one another. *You. No, you.* Finally, the employee cleared his throat. "Can I ask you something?" he said, face turning red with embarrassment.

"Sure," I said, figuring it had something to do with work.

"You always come out smiling," he began, faltering. "And every time you're in there, I can feel the vibrations from all the way out here. Can I ask..." He hesitated again.

Needless to say, I laughed and explained, my cheeks turning perhaps a little bit pink. From then on, I made sure to put the pump on the floor, where it made a whole lot less buzz around the office.

# One Too Many

My pressure-cooker job as a business consultant frequently included all-nighters, but it did nothing to prepare me for the soul-destroying sleep deprivation of breastfeeding infant twins.

One night, my husband was working late; I fell asleep after a seemingly endless day of breastfeeding two babies. After awhile, I half awakened and staggered down the hall to the babies' room to return whomever I had been breastfeeding (I really couldn't keep track sometimes) to the crib they shared. In my sleep-deprived stupor, I looked into the crib and counted one baby, two babies... then shrieked as I realized I had very carefully carried my left breast down the hall.

I am happy to say that my left breast no longer resembles either of my children.

# Live Sculpture

When my daughter was about five months old, we went to the Museum of Contemporary Art in Chicago with our new mothers' group. Each week, our gang of new moms and babies got together for an outing of some kind.

It was early afternoon as we strolled through the galleries, and one by one the babies started to fuss. There was a very long glass bench in the middle of the large exhibit hall, so the ten of us (five moms plus five hungry babies) sat down to take a nursing break—three of us facing one way and two the other.

Within moments we began to attract attention. The museum visitors thought we were a modern art installation! Several art patrons milled around us, intently watching this "live sculpture" with serious looks on their faces. The babies nursed happily while we moms stifled our giggles.

Nursing as art!

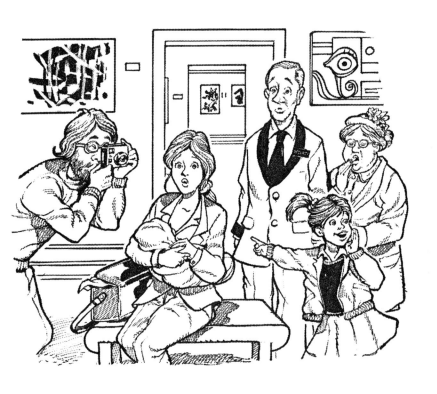

# Sock It to Ya

One weekend I was nursing my son when my husband thought it would be funny to tease him by pretending that he was nursing from me, too. I thought it was pretty funny until my usually sweet son became fed up. He started to frown very deeply, but my husband didn't notice.

The next thing I knew, my son had socked my husband in the eye *hard*! My husband pouted, but my son turned back into an angel.

Let this be a lesson to others: Never tease a breastfeeding baby.

# Wardrobe Malfunction

Nowadays, you might label it a "wardrobe malfunction." When it happened to me, it was just plain embarrassing—that is, until I saw the humor in it.

My first baby was a healthy, good-size boy. Breast-feeding had gone smoothly at first, but now my four-month-old was refusing to nurse.

After phoning La Leche League and speaking to their local leader, I decided to attend one of their meetings. I had imagined a formal lecture-style setting: a room with folding chairs in rows facing a speaker. As I entered the meeting, I saw about twenty-five women with their babies, sitting on couches, chairs, and the carpet. There were babies nursing everywhere I looked! None of my friends had babies yet, nor had any of my family members nursed their babies. In fact, I had never actually seen anyone else nurse a baby. I was elated to be among women who thought like I did.

After talking about my problem with others, we moved into the kitchen for a snack. I sat in a chair, my baby now nursing contentedly. I thought about the cause of my baby's frequent refusal to nurse during the last few weeks: My husband and I had just bought a house—our first one—and I was nervous and reluctant to move. Emotionally I wasn't ready for any more changes. Our baby must have sensed my distress.

While I continued to nurse and reflect on what I could do to remedy the situation, the door opened and two men walked in. My first reaction was to cover up; I was self-conscious about my large breasts. Big to start with, they felt enormous during those first few months of nursing. (When I walked through a door, my breasts came through seconds sooner than the rest of me.) I tried to pull my sweater over the breast my baby wasn't attached to. It wouldn't move! It was caught in my bra's cup closure, and no amount of tugging would release it.

Seeing how flustered I was, a woman beside me explained that the two men were "just dads of breastfed babies." But before she could finish speaking, I had jumped up and started to run to the bathroom. I was hunched over, head down, baby at my breast, flying toward the bathroom. To make matters worse, this awkward position put a strain on my pants' zipper. Too vain to wear my better-fitting maternity slacks, I had left the top button undone on my pre-pregnancy pants. I felt as if all eyes were on me as my slacks slipped down my backside.

My pants fell completely down just after I burst through the bathroom door. I shuffled over to the toilet and sat down. Reviewing what had just happened, I felt so embarrassed! I pictured how I must have looked with my pants falling off during my mad scramble to hide. Viewing it from that perspective, I thought to myself, "Hey, this is actually funny." Instead of crying, I had a good laugh at myself, the first I'd had in weeks.

# Get the Pacifier

I was catching up on some calls one evening, so I left my baby son in my husband's care. I had just nursed him, but he was still fussy. My husband had had some difficulty handling him before, so we'd discussed several ways for my husband to soothe him. One surefire trick was to use a pacifier, which we always called a "binkie."

Because I was on the phone, my husband called to my older son and asked him to "get the pacifier." My older kids liked to take turns on what they called "bink duty," in which one child was responsible for locating and popping the binkie into the baby's mouth. Having not heard the word *pacifier* before, "get the pacifier" didn't register with my son. After receiving only a puzzled look, my husband explained, "You know, those things the baby sucks on when he's trying to sleep?"

A light bulb seemed to suddenly illuminate above my son's head. He jumped up, ran into the kitchen—where I was on the phone with our Sunday School coordinator—and shouted, "Mom! Dad wants to see your boobs!"

# Diagnosis

There I was, sitting on a hard chair in an examination room, waiting yet again to see the family doctor. It seemed so unnecessary to drag my tiny two-week-old back here for a third time, just so she could be weighed (and coughed on by every person in the waiting room).

After a wail they could probably hear across town, I fumbled to undo my bra strap. Would I ever be able to do this in public without feeling clumsy? My daughter latched on to my nipple like a hungry wolf cub. Her appetite was as ferocious as her temper.

Of course, the long-awaited doctor appeared only moments after I had gotten her nicely settled in. Plucking my contented babe from my breast, he cradled her in his arms. He met my eyes briefly before we both looked down to watch my milk come in. Sitting nearly three feet away from him did little to control the damage: From belly to toe, he had been soaked in breast milk.

He smirked. "So I take it you aren't having much trouble with milk flow."

# Reckless Driving

How many moms want to breastfeed, but have jobs that just don't work in their favor? I had that problem, but I was determined to breastfeed, regardless of my situation. I'm an account executive who has no privacy and no extra time. So when I found a breast pump with an adapter for my car's cigarette lighter, I was in heaven.

My first week back to work was wonderful. I took three breaks to run out to the car and pump, and I got six to eight ounces at every pumping—more than enough to keep my daughter happy. But the second week was a challenge. After three months away, I had to play catch up with all my clients. On Friday, I scheduled two appointments too close together. I was pinched for time. And I was engorged. When I say engorged, I mean my melons were ripe, and *ouch*, they hurt.

So I did the only thing I could: I brought the cow into the barn, so to speak. I hooked myself to the pump, then put the car in drive. I headed down the highway, being careful not to pass any trucks or vehicles that might have passengers who could see into my car. The gentle *whoosh whoosh* of the pump was playing along with the radio, and I was doing fine until the big rig I was behind started to slow down. I had to pass, so I put the pedal to the metal and did it as fast as I could.

After I passed the rig, I saw a car come flying up behind me. I hoped it wouldn't pass me and see me pumping. Well, I got my wish. It didn't pass me. Instead, there were flashing blue lights in my rearview mirror. Talk about your heart stopping and your milk freezing up! This couldn't be happening! ➡️

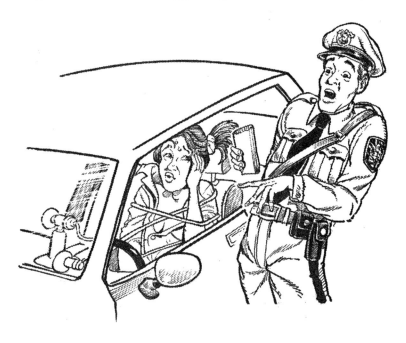

I set the bottles in the passenger seat and tried to unhook the pump while I pulled off the road. I didn't have time to adjust myself, so I must have looked awfully interesting as the officer approached the car. He looked over my shoulder, asked for my license and registration, and started his "Do you know why..." speech.

I tried to collect myself and think of a good story, but I decided the truth would be the best approach. As I explained about being late for a meeting, I could tell I wasn't impressing him. But when I added the breastfeeding part, I saw a little smirk on his face, then a full grin that led right into a foot-stomping laugh. He told me his wife breastfed his son, and he thought it was great that I was so devoted to the cause.

I didn't get off *too* easily. He said I was driving recklessly and gave me a good scolding and a warning, but no ticket. I haven't attempted to pump and drive since.

# Fix-It Man

I was sitting across the room from my three-year-old son when my breasts started to leak. My son, who loves to play fix-it man, heard me say, "Oh no, I'm leaking!"

He answered, "What's leaking? I'm a plumber—I can fix it!"

When I told him my milk was leaking, he said, "Oh, I'm not *that* kind of plumber!"

# When You Think You're Prepared...

L ike most older moms-to-be, I read everything I could get my hands on about pregnancy, childbirth, and childcare. And I was determined to nurse, so I read everything I could find about breastfeeding, too.

I had a fantasy in my mind of when my baby would arrive: My husband, David, would hold my hand, dab sweat from my forehead, and whisper encouraging words in my ear. The midwife would croon, "One more push, sugar," which would be a breeze since I'd Kegeled three hours a day for seven months. Then into the delivery room a perfect, pink boy or girl would emerge and take right to my breast, nursing lustily while David captured the whole thing on video.

Instead I awoke in my eighth month in a puddle of blood. We drove frantically to the hospital, where I was knocked out and given an emergency cesarean section. At least that's what I was told several hours later when I awoke in a drug-induced stupor. But my lactation counselor was there, so at least the breastfeeding part of my fantasy could come true. The counselor helped me arrange Haley at my breast, but the drugs were so strong, I wavered in and out of consciousness, finally conking out, dead to the world. "No problem," my lactation guru announced. She nestled Haley to my breast and told my husband, "Here! Hold this." Then she left.

The pictures of Haley's first breastfeeding experience look nothing like the ones in the books. I am passed out, head flopped to one side, spittle drooling from my mouth. David is holding Haley with a befuddled won't-someone-help-me look and, sure enough, Haley is nursing.

After reading and memorizing all those books on breastfeeding, I have to live with the fact that my husband got to breastfeed our baby before I did.

# The Head Nipple Inspector

·  ·  ·  ·  ·  ·  ·  ·  ·  ·  ·  ·  ·  ·  ·  ·  ·  ·  ·  ·  ·  ·  ·  ·  ·

Seven months into my pregnancy, I found myself at a La Leche League meeting with my friend Yvonne, the reigning queen of breastfeeding and the person I was determined to dethrone.

Yvonne had nursed her three children over six straight years. She whipped her breasts out whenever and wherever, donated her milk to the children's hospital, and raved about a nursing support group called the La Leche League.

"You'll have to come to a meeting," she said when I told her I was pregnant.

"I'd love to. What do you do?"

"Oh, we learn nursing techniques. The proper latch, the football hold."

"The football hold?"

"You hold the baby like a football under your arm. It works for some. I prefer the cradle hold. I can help you with it."

"I'm sure I can figure it out. What else do you do?"

"Well," she said, "they'll probably want to inspect your nipples."

"Inspect my nipples?"

"Yeah, you know, to see if they're inverted or something else that will cause you problems."

"Inspect my nipples?"

"Let me know when it's good for you."

I wondered if it would ever be good for me.

Yvonne and I had been best friends in high school. We did everything together. Our periods were synchronized; we lost our virginity on the same night. We planned to marry best friends, live next door to each other in a cul-de-sac, and have best-friend children.

But Yvonne beat me to the altar, the cul-de-sac, and the maternity ward. We were still best friends, but she had the kids and the other mothers at La Leche League. Meanwhile, I kept basal temperature charts and elevated my hips after intercourse. And then one morning, there were two stripes in the window of my Clear Blue Easy test, and I was on my way to motherhood and a meeting with a nipple inspector.

At my first meeting, a woman took a seat at the front of the group. She was tall and wore jeans and sandals. I imagined she had hairy armpits and was a vegetarian.

"That's her," Yvonne said.

"Who?"

"The Head Nipple Inspector."

She had big, hardworking hands with sturdy fingers. I looked at my reflection in the window. I looked poised, confident; a woman with child-bearing hips and noninverted nipples. "Bring it on," I thought. Yvonne patted my tummy and winked.

"We should get going," The Head Nipple Inspector said. "But before we start, let's go around the room and introduce ourselves. I understand," she said, nodding toward me and rubbing her fingertips together (warming them, perhaps), "there's a first-timer in our midst."

Everyone leaned forward, looking at my face and tits, and smiling in anticipation of my initiation.

"Let's start from this end," the Inspector said, pointing to a woman at the start of the semicircle.

Introductions were made. They got closer and closer to me. I had to pee and I thought, "I'll get up, go to the bathroom, and they'll never notice." But then it was my turn. The Inspector walked toward me, her hand extended, reaching for my chest. I quickly stood, closed my eyes, unhooked my bra, and lifted my smock, exposing myself to the Head Nipple Inspector.

"Well," she said, clearing her throat, "you're going to fit right in."

I opened my eyes. "You might want to do this yourself," she said, as she handed me a "My Name Is" sticker.

I did up the clasp on my bra, smoothed out my shirt, and sat down.

"What were you doing?" Yvonne asked, laughing softly.

"You told me they'd inspect my nipples." I whispered, then laughed as well, covering my face.

"I was just kidding!"

"Oh, now you tell me."

"Well," Yvonne said, "if it's any consolation, they look great. Really, better than mine. I had such trouble to begin with, but you've got those eraser heads going on. You're a natural."

"Do you think?"

Yvonne nodded and raised her eyebrows. I don't think she even felt the crown leave her head.

# How to Feed Quintuplets

As much as my husband and I tried to prepare our two young boys for the fact that their new baby sister would be getting her food from Mommy's boobs, they still had a million questions.

But one night while at my mother's house, my six-year-old proved he at least understood the concept. We were watching a story on TV about a woman who had had quintuplets. My son looked at my mother and said, "Man, she's gonna need a lot of boobs to feed those babies!"

# Keeping Count

As a hospital nurse, I once spent a lot of time caring for a brand-new mother and her baby. When I left them for the night, I told the mom to leave me a note in the crib, saying how long her baby had nursed and how many wet and dirty diapers the infant had had.

When I picked up the infant for morning lab work the next day, the mom was still asleep. In the crib was a note that said the baby had had one wet diaper, two messy diapers, and approximately 784 sucks.

That poor mom, thinking she had to count each suck at every feeding instead of just estimating how many *minutes* the baby had nursed. The relief on her face was priceless!

# My Deer
# Little Jessica

Years ago, before I had my own children, I honed my parenting skills by baby-sitting my cousin's nine-month-old, Jessica.

My cousin, toting a Ralph Lauren diaper bag armed with enough disposable diapers to wallpaper the living room, babbled baby-care instructions at me before leaving Jessica at my home in the country: "Here's her 'bwankie,' and don't forget she loves books. This one's her favorite. Oh, and I'll put her bottle in the fridge. It has a breast-simulating nipple so she'll think she's actually nursing. I just expressed the milk an hour ago, so it should be fine in the fridge until I get home. I'll be back by 5:00, or when my breasts explode from engorgement—whichever comes first."

"Bye, bye, Mommy!" I babbled in my best baby voice. I scooped the pristine cherub from her mother.

How difficult could it be to care for a nine-month-old for a couple hours? After all, I earned good grades in college. This should be a cinch. Then Jessica made an explosive sound from somewhere below her bellybutton. Let the baby-sitting begin!

I spent the rest of the afternoon playing with Jessica. We played peekaboo. We read books. I introduced

Jessica to my dog, cat, and the injured white-tailed fawn I was caring for.

"This baby-sitting thing is way too fun," I confided to Jessica at naptime. She stuck a fat fist into her drooling mouth and waited with hungry eyes for me to serve her before-nap appetizer. I retrieved her bottle from the refrigerator and popped the nipple into her open mouth.

Gulp, gulp, gulp.... The baby's eyes grew wide as she consumed the contents of the pink bottle.

"How's that, sweetie?" I cooed. My Child Development 101 textbook had stressed the correlation between verbal stimulation and cognitive development in infants. "Do you love Mommy's milky?"

Gulp, gulp, gulp.... Jessica thrust her head forward and back like an excited chicken. She seemed to have some difficulty swallowing the milk—must have been the unfamiliar breast-simulating nipple.

Having never looked closely at breast milk before, I was impressed. "Wow, this milk is substantial! How could a woman's breasts produce liquid so thick?" I wondered aloud. I reasoned that breast milk *is* Mother

39

Nature's perfect food. Who was I to question her divine plan?

Just then the front door opened. "I'm home!" sang my cousin, hurrying in, refreshed from her reprieve. "How's my... AAAAAHHHHHHH! What are you feeding my child?"

Little Jessica sat up, clumps of milk—possibly regurgitated—clinging to her chin. "What *is* this stuff?" my cousin gasped, yanking the bottle from her daughter's drooling mouth.

"It's breast milk! Don't you recognize your own body fluid?" I retorted.

"I...I did not produce that," stammered Jessica's mother.

"Well, if it's not breast milk, then it must be...oh my gosh...concentrated deer formula!"

Holy hooters.

Apparently, in my zeal to play surrogate mother, I had grabbed the fawn's bottle from the fridge and fed it to one very hungry baby. A quick call to Poison Control reassured us: "The baby may experience a little diarrhea, some fussiness, but deer formula is essentially concentrated goat's milk, not considered poisonous to

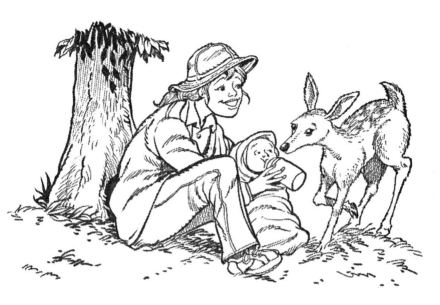

infants. However, if you notice any unusual neck elongation or suspicious bleating...*baaaaa!*" I hung up.

Later that week, my cousin called to give me an update on Jessica's condition. "She seems fine. No vomiting or diarrhea; happy as can be. But you know, she just doesn't seem as...motivated to drink expressed breast milk. It's funny—I think she actually preferred the deer food!"

Since the Dehydrated Deer Formula Incident, I have given birth to and nursed six children of my own. I have to admit it, though: Whenever I reach in the refrigerator to feed my baby a bottle of expressed breast milk, I always think of my "deer" little Jessica.

# The Pumping Police

When I returned to work after maternity leave, I was a little anxious about using my breast pump, but I was determined to continue nursing. Because I was on the road all the time for work, I had plenty of privacy to pump in my car. Or did I?

When it was time to pump one day, I found a quiet parking lot near the beach. As I set up my gear, I saw several people hiking by, so I decided to put up my car shades for more privacy.

I was happily pumping away when I looked in my rearview mirror and, to my horror, saw a police officer quickly approaching my car. He must have been suspicious of the blocked windows and someone's silhouette clearly inside. I tried to adjust myself quickly, but spilled my liquid gold all over as he began to bang on my window.

I initially ignored him as I attempted to get settled, but he banged louder and yelled, "What's going on in there?"

I rolled down my window and, feeling rather frustrated, blurted, "If you really want to know, I'm using my breast pump!"

The police officer retreated quickly with a horrified look on his face. As he walked away, he spoke into his shoulder walkie-talkie. To this day, I wish I could have heard what he said to his dispatcher!

# A Little-Known
# Breastfeeding Benefit

I was at the hairdresser's with my two young daughters and my baby son. I'd been lucky to find a one-hour parking spot directly in front of the shop, which was in a bustling part of the city.

Just as the hairdresser was about to finish cutting my second daughter's hair, my son woke up, so I breastfed him. We were getting comfortable together, having a lovely feed when I noticed a parking inspector examining my car. Looking at my watch, I realized with shock and horror that I'd been parked for over an hour. I was about to get a parking ticket.

I raced out to the car, apologizing profusely, trying to explain that I'd be only a few more minutes. When the parking inspector glanced up, his jaw dropped and his eyes looked like they would pop out of his head. At that moment, I realized I'd run into the middle of the busy shopping strip with my son still firmly attached to my breast and feeding away without missing a beat.

The parking inspector apologized profusely to *me* and was happy to let me finish feeding before moving the car.

We all know there are many advantages to breast-feeding—avoiding a parking ticket just isn't one of the most publicized!

# An Areola Never Forgets

I had breast and lip enlargements done at the same time, about two years before I got pregnant. The doctor took scar tissue from my areola and placed it inside my lips.

After having my daughter, I tried for three days to nurse her. Not only were my breasts getting bigger, but so were my lips! Bigger and bigger, to the point that I couldn't talk, could barely eat, and had to go around with my hand over my mouth because my lips were so huge! I told a doctor about it and asked if he thought my lips were trying to lactate. He laughed and said it was quite possible that the tissue had retained its memory.

It was a hard decision to make, but I quit nursing, and now my lips are fine again. Lactating lips—who'd have thought?

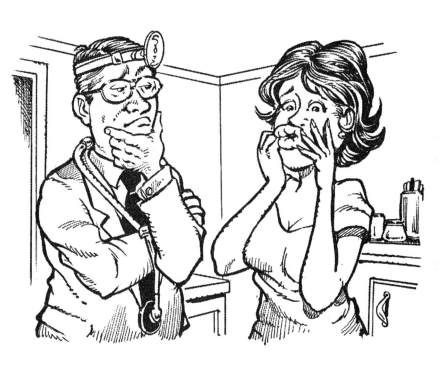

# Naturally

After baby number one stopped breastfeeding and was into peas and macaroni and cheese as her staple diet, along came baby number two. At some point, two-and-a-half-year-old Emma noticed that baby Jared was not drinking from a sippy cup or even a bottle.

"What's he doing, Mommy?"

"Drinking milk."

"Did I do that?"

"Yes." I watched her tiny face. Her forehead scrunched in concentration. What was she thinking? After careful consideration, Emma decided to leave breastfeeding to her baby brother. But she stored the memory away, ready for the ideal moment to let him in on the secret. That day arrived three years later.

"You used to do it." Emma sounded like a determined but frustrated teacher, explaining the obvious yet again to her class.

"Me did not." Jared shook his head, his voice indignant. At three, he was ready to argue with his five-year-old sister, especially when he *knew* she was wrong.

"Did too."

"Mommy!"

Feet pounded up to my bedroom where I stood, folding laundry. For a second I considered hiding in the laundry hamper. But they were too quick for me.

Putting her hands on her hips, Emma glared at me. "Mommy, tell Jared."

"Tell him what?"

"Tell him about your bra."

"What? This?" I dangled the undergarment in front of her.

"No." She pointed at my chest. "Those."

"These? What about them?" I threw a pair of socks onto Emma's pile, but looked longingly at the hamper. If only I had jumped.

"You used to feed Jared with them, right?" She continued to point accusingly at my chest.

"I breastfed you, too."

"Really?" She raised an eyebrow. Her hand dismissed the idea. "I know you fed him milk with them because I saw you. When he was a baby."

"That's right."

"Told you." She smiled triumphantly at Jared. "I'm right."

For a moment Jared stared at me, his eyes wide. Then he shrugged a very manly shrug. "That's okay, Mommy." He hugged me, patting my back.

"Uh, thanks, Jared." Was he trying to comfort me? "It's normal to breastfeed, by the way, and it's healthy. Humans do it, and so do lots of animals."

What else could I say? Breastfeeding seemed like an alien concept to my children, despite the fact I'd nursed them both for months. Maybe I could show them it was normal. But how? I didn't have any photos or video of me breastfeeding them. Did I have a friend who was nursing? Maybe if we sat long enough at the family room in the mall, my children would witness breastfeeding. Desperate, I wondered if there were any newborn puppies or kittens at the animal shelter....

It was suddenly quiet. Too quiet. Where were my children? Folding the final towel, I decided I'd better find them. I could hear whispers in Jared's room. Curious, I stood by the door. "This is the teddy's baby, Jared," I heard.

I poked my head in. "What are you two doing?"

"Shh, Mommy," Jared whispered. "Babies."

"Babies?"

"Yes, Mommy." Emma nodded at her bear, a little plush dog nuzzled to its chest. "The babies are drinking, and then they're going to sleep. You have to be quiet." She put her finger to her lips.

There, on Jared's bed, were stuffed animals nursing other stuffed animals, indiscriminant of species. Dogs nursed cats, teddy bears mothered monkeys.

"Oh. Okay." I whispered, and tiptoed away.

My children had grappled with the profundities of human life, and instinctively they reenacted the experience with their own babies. Naturally.

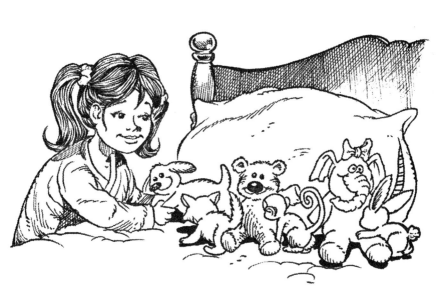

# All Pads Are Not Created Equal

When my husband, daughter, and I were invited to visit my sister for the weekend, I jumped at the chance. She'd breastfed four kids and I figured I could pick up some tips. (Plus snag a nap or two, while we were there.) Everything went fine until Saturday evening, when we dressed for church.

An overabundance of milk had never been a problem for me, so I hadn't thought to pack the box of breast pads they'd given me at the hospital. But when I looked at the sheer, white blouse I planned to wear, I realized there was a chance that I might be standing in the pew with two wet stains on the front of my blouse for God and everybody to see. There wasn't time to run to the drugstore, so my sister conceived the brilliant idea of cutting two minipads into little ovals and fitting them inside my nursing bra. She figured a pad was a pad, right?

My Kotex-turned-breast pads were a lifesaver when, halfway through the service, my breasts decided it was party time. As the breast milk soaked the pads but not my shirt, I smiled at how clever we'd been. How wrong I was!

What we hadn't considered was that the pads were scented, and the perfume covered my breasts. When poor Haley woke to nurse that night, she didn't recognize the funny taste. And so began one of the longest nights of my life.

She'd latch on to nurse just long enough to trigger my milk production. Then she'd pull away and cry. My breasts would expand. She'd latch on again, more milk would let down, she'd pull away and cry, my breasts would grow even BIGGER. Latch, letdown, pull away and cry, grow. Repeat.

I didn't want to wake my sister, so I sat there lactating and hurting until dawn. Haley finally wore herself out and fell asleep hungry and miserable. Sleeping was not an option for me. By the time my sister woke up, I could barely stand the pain in my breasts. She got me into a hot shower, where it soon looked as though I had two whale spouts shooting from my chest. It was hours before we put two and two together and figured out what we'd done.

From then on, I *always* packed breast pads.

# The Evil Twin Goes Shopping

When my son Gavin was about six weeks old, the kiddos and I were in Wal-Mart doing the usual family shopping. The baby was in the sling, hooked up and nursing. Feeling confident, as usual, that all was well on the nursing front (that is, I was appropriately covered), I pushed the shopping cart through the children's department. There I was approached by a woman who was very enthusiastic about seeing a newborn...or two.

She ran up to me and excitedly asked if I had twins. I said cautiously, "No, why do you ask?" as a sinking feeling washed over me. We simultaneously looked down at the baby in the sling and realized that the other "head" she was seeing was my big, ol', pasty-white boob! My shirt was up under my armpit and, boy, did it look as if there were two babies in my sling! She quickly looked up at me, screeched that she was sorry, and took off running to the shoe department.

Feeling ridiculous and trying not to have an accident from my intense laughter, I gathered up my son's "evil twin" and returned to shopping. It was so funny and embarrassing, I'm sure the store's security folks watch the tape from time to time for a good laugh.

# Rude Awakening

When my oldest daughter, Claire, was a newborn, I was a nervous wreck. Breastfeeding seemed natural and went pretty smoothly, but I was terribly paranoid about SIDS. I read everything I could find on the subject and discovered that dressing babies in sleepers wards off blanket suffocation. So I dutifully went out and bought warm sleepers for Claire.

But I still had a dilemma: I was breastfeeding Claire at night and found it easiest to keep her by my side so I could go back to sleep while she nursed. I needed covers for myself, but I was afraid to cover her. So as soon as she fell asleep after nursing, I scooted down the bed so she was by my head. I could be under the covers without having her under them, too.

This trick worked until one night, I woke up with a terrible shooting pain, as if someone were tearing my lips off. I opened my eyes and was startled to find my little angel latched on to my upper lip!

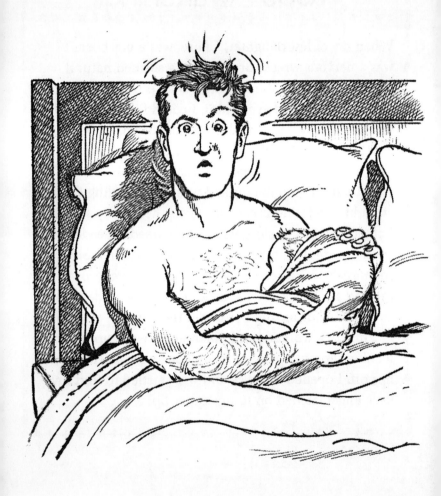

# Have Nipple, Will Nurse

The funniest breastfeeding experience I ever had was when my daughter, Emily, was only three days old, although technically it didn't happen to me.

Since her birth, Emily had been pretty much nursing constantly. That particular morning, I had to go to the bathroom before she was done. I thrust her at my husband and asked him to take over. He happily laid her belly to belly on his chest. Before too long, Emily began rooting around. She very quickly found what she was looking for.

I returned to the room to his screaming. He was lifting her up and yelping. With every lift, her head went down and his chest expanded. Seems that my little girl didn't care whose nipple she got into her newborn mouth. Of course, I hadn't bothered to explain to my husband how to unlatch a nursing baby, as I never thought he would need to know! I just stood there laughing until he finally lifted her high enough to force her to let go.

He wouldn't hold our little Jaws without wearing a shirt for a long time after that.

# What Husbands Don't Know Won't Hurt Them

●●●●●●●●●●●●●●●●●●●●●●●●●

When my son, Eytan, was five months old, my extended family decided to have a huge weekend reunion at a campground.

"I'm not going," my husband, John, grumbled. "I always sleep badly, we eat crap from cans, and I can't get a decent cup of coffee. Besides, we have a new baby!"

"He'll cuddle up to me in my sleeping bag with my breast on tap all the time. He'll love it!" I knew I'd love it, too. It would be the first time my whole family had been together in over ten years. I figured I could make a pot of John's beloved coffee ahead of time and reheat it over the campfire. (Don't shudder, coffee drinkers. This was the best I could come up with.) So I argued and pushed and pleaded, and in the end we went.

It was a glorious campsite. I introduced Eytan to lake water in the day and cuddled him by the fire at night. The family meals were delicious, and John smacked his lips appreciatively over his coffee the first morning. All went smoothly until the second day.

I got up first and bustled about making a fire and heating up the coffee, with Eytan lying on a blanket and gurgling at the trees. Then disaster struck. As soon as I opened the icebox, I could smell the carton of milk. I tasted it in blind hope, and spat the revolting stuff out all over my chin.

What to do? John always took his coffee with milk! Then Eytan burped. I looked down as a stream of milk trickled out of his mouth, and he looked back with interest at the milky curds still decorating my own chin. I had an idea.

Positioning my breast over the steaming cup, I aimed a stream of milk into the black coffee. First one breast, then the other. It took quite a lot of milk to lighten it to its usual color, and there were fat bubbles floating on the surface, but I hoped John wouldn't notice in the gloomy interior of the tent.

"Coffee time," I said brightly. "Served in your sleeping bag as a special treat."

John sat up and sipped his coffee. "Mmm," he said. "Delicious."

# The Titty Fairy

Three days in the hospital after an emergency cesarean section, I was still drugged and more asleep than awake. After one seemingly innocent nap, I awoke to discover that the Titty Fairy had paid me a visit: My breasts had quadrupled in size and were exploding out of the top of my nursing gown.

I was afraid to move. All I could do was whisper to my sister dozing in a chair, "Psst, Denise, get the camera. Quick, get the camera!"

My husband, David, was home taking a shower, and I wasn't even sure if I was awake or dreaming, so I had to get a photo preserving the day Mom had bodacious ta-tas, for our family history.

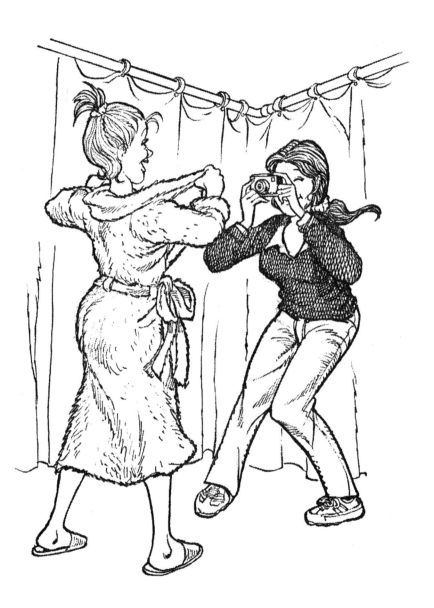

# Party Girl

My breasts look so fabulous, I can't stop staring at them in the mirror. Since having my baby, Drew, four months ago, I've been padding around the house in my disgusting maternity shirts, but tomorrow night, that ends. I have a party to go to, one that will be filled with all my childless friends, and I am going to look amazing—thanks in part to my new silicone breast shields.

In the months since the baby was born, I've sprung several leaks with my dual set of Old Faithfuls. When I bother to wear a nursing bra, I double up the nursing pads. I end up with these weird, migrating lumpy bumps on my chest. I sometimes try to tape them down with surgical tape, and I have red Xs from the adhesive on my skin to prove it. But I recently found out about these silicone breast shields that are nothing short of a miracle. They are thin and self-sticking and leak proof (or at least that's what the package says).

In honor of my fancy new breast shields, I have been rooting through my dresser like an archaeologist on a dig. I burrow past the frumpy granny underwear, past the hideous nursing bras with their torturous snap contraptions, down through layers of forgotten lingerie. I have found evidence of thongs. Cute matching sets of bras and panties. A garter belt. Stockings. *Stockings*, I tell you!

But the girl who owned this stuff was a lot thinner than I am. Granted, she did not have a beautiful baby, but she did have an exquisite silky designer bra with a swirly pattern and no function or purpose other than to make her look amazing. It's actually one of the larger BC (Before Child) bras I can find. I blow out all the air from my lungs and try it on. Amazingly, I am able to catch the largest setting after only a few tries. I gingerly let go, expecting the whole thing to spring off my body, ricochet around the room, and break a potted plant. But miraculously it holds. And although my cups runneth over, I look freaking fabulous. It really takes my breath away, although that could just be the band cutting into my ribcage.

Later at the party, it's obvious that my efforts were all worth it. There are tiny white lights strung in the trees, tiki torches on the porch. My husband, Rob, is lolling around by the DJ table, shooting smoldering looks my way. It was hard for us to leave Drew with his grandparents (between us we have three cell phones and a beeper, and are poised to race out the door at a moment's notice), but for the moment time is standing still. I wink at Rob over my best friend Lisa's shoulder. I feel a sudden rush of love, and it actually feels like pins and needles up and down my arms.

"Jeez, I have all these superintense 'new mom' hormones. I feel crazed with love all the time," I mutter. Not to mention I am having a little trouble breathing from the constant pressure on my chest. "I can't even watch the news at night without bawling."

"Stop watching the news! You just need to watch more *Teletubbies*," says Lisa with an evil grin. "By the way, you are lookin' good tonight!" she says. "Foxy. Hot!" She licks her finger and makes a sizzle sound.

"Yeah...speaking of hot, is it like a million degrees here all of the sudden, or what?" My hormone rush has left me feeling flushed and dizzy, still tingly, and kind of...wet. "Oh, my God."

"What?" Her eyes widen. "Oh, my God," she echoes. "You spilled your, um, your shirt is, um, you have—"

I cut her off. "No kidding. My freaking stupid milk just let down, and my freaking stupid breast shields are a freaking stupid disaster!" My chest is burning hot and wet and slippery, and the milk seems to be leaking around the breast shields in perfect rings. Somehow we make it to the bathroom, and I immediately yank off the horrible bra and dump it in a heap on the floor. There's a bright red band that goes all the way around my ribcage, and I massage it tenderly. I feel the pins and needles again, and milk starts gently spraying out of one of my breasts. I hear a soft knock on the door.

"Hey, it's me," Rob says. "Let me come in."

"Sure," I say bitterly. "Hey, you want some milk?"

He swears no one even noticed The Great Milk Run. I am crumpled up in the passenger seat on the way home, shivering and cranking the heat. My breasts are throbbing. "What's your deal?" he says. "It's almost eighty degrees in here."

"I know," I moan. "Just turn up the seat heater, will you?"

"Yeah, I turned it up the last time you asked me. It's on ten already."

"Well, turn it up *more*."

The capstone experience of my wonderful night out is getting mastitis, a direct result of wearing constricting undergarments. Rob has to take care of Drew pretty much on his own, although I still breastfeed him. My fever goes up to 104 degrees, but the higher my temperature gets, the colder I feel. At the height of my fever I'm using a heating pad, electric blanket, and down comforter all at the same time and I'm still not warm enough.

I have to ask myself, was it all worth it? Yes. Yes! A million times yes. All the pain was worth it for my five minutes of supreme hotness. (But you won't be seeing me in that deathtrap bra again any time soon.)

# Nurse

When my son, Toby, was about eighteen months old, he was walking and learning to speak, but still nursing. I firmly believed he should continue to nurse as long as he wanted and did nothing to discourage him.

My mother, visiting for two weeks from Connecticut, had other ideas. She would chastise Toby whenever he wanted to nurse, saying, "You're a big boy now. You're too old to be nursing." Like many people, she felt if he was old enough to ask, he was too old to nurse.

Toby, however, was in no rush to give up that special time he and I shared. One day when we had settled into the rocking chair for a naptime nurse, my mom came into the room and told Toby he should get into his bed like a big boy.

Toby climbed down from my lap. Without a word, he walked to my mother, took her hand, and led her out of the bedroom. When she was just outside the room, he shut the door on her, then walked back and climbed up into my lap. He looked at me, smiled, and said, "Nurse?"

From the other side of the door, I could hear an exclamation of surprise, then muffled laughter as my mother realized what Toby had done.

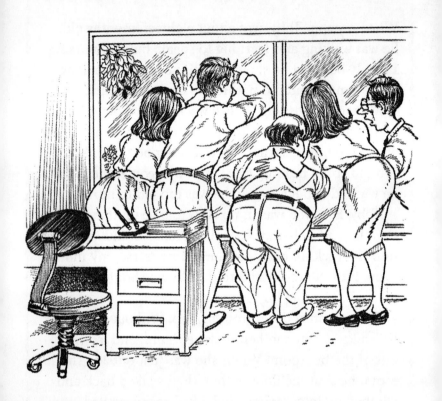

# Suburban Suspect

There was nowhere at work to use my breast pump, so I had to resort to pumping in the back of my Suburban, which had very dark tinted windows. I eventually got so used to this routine that I didn't even think of what it might look like to others: A young woman climbing into the back of an SUV, staying there for fifteen minutes, then straightening her clothing upon getting out.

I also didn't notice the looks from other employees who worked within my building. That is, until I was climbing out after a nice, relaxing session of pumping to classical music, and I happened to glance up and see an audience in the window. I suddenly realized that a rumor must have gotten around these poor, boring offices about questionable business going on in the parking lot (the word *nooner* came to mind).

When I went to pump the next day, I posted a very bold and readable sign on the Suburban's window that stated: "Sorry to disappoint you, but I am merely lactating."

After that, the onlookers went back to work.

# They Never Outgrow That

My husband, Larry, and I are known as the family "granolas," and some of the things we do make our loving family members shake their heads. For example, they think it's a bit strange that I continue to nurse my almost two-year-old son, Paul. So to avoid the teasing and eye rolling, I don't nurse in front of them much.

When our oven suddenly quit working one day, Larry called his brother, Don, for advice. Don was nearby, so he agreed to stop and check it out. He was with his wife, her sister, his brother-in-law, and a friend of theirs, and they were all coming with Don to our home.

When our guests arrived, we split by gender. The men gathered in the kitchen to do voodoo on the stove, while the women chitchatted in the living room. Paul was content to stay in the kitchen watching his daddy use tools—until something happened and he came out of the kitchen crying and looking for Mommy's comfort.

I probably would have picked him up and nursed him right then, but I didn't know these other people at all. Besides wanting to avoid the teasing, I didn't want Paul to expose my breasts in front of strangers. He can't stand having his face covered while nursing, and he frequently pushes my shirt out of his way.

I tried to head him off by picking him up and putting him over my shoulder. Nothing doing. He pushed his little body off my shoulder and lay himself horizontally in my arms, screeching. I still had hopes of calming him down and continuing to visit, so I offered him a bite of chicken. That's when he really made his wishes known. He pressed his open hands on my breasts and slid his palms all over my chest, then tried to pull up my shirt, shouting, "Booby, booby, booby, booby!"

By now the guys had finished in the kitchen, and everyone was being entertained by Paul's antics. I stood to go into the bedroom and nurse him. I opened my mouth to excuse myself and thank everyone for coming over, when one of the male guests put the scene in perspective. With a smile, he said, "We never outgrow that."

# Excuse Me, Dear...

I had just started venturing out of the house after the birth of my second child when I decided to stock up on groceries. I headed into the grocery store with my toddler, Olyvia, and my baby, Elyas.

Everything went pretty smoothly at first. I put the baby into the baby seat on the cart and was gathering the items I needed. After about fifteen minutes, though, Elyas started fussing, and Olyvia started throwing random things into the cart. While I tried to put back the unnecessary items, Elyas continued to fuss. I knew I needed to nurse him. The tension was building, and I was really starting to feel the pressure of being an inexperienced new mother of two!

Unexpectedly, I felt a gentle tap on my shoulder. I turned to hear a little old lady say, "Excuse me, dear, but your milk is leaking."

I froze. I was devastated! The idea of having two huge wet spots on my shirt sent me into panic and embarrassment. I looked down at my blouse, thinking the baby's fussing caused me to let down all over my shirt.

As I feverishly continued searching for obvious signs, the lady said again, "Honey, your milk is leaking."

I started to cry and in sheer frustration said, "Where? Where do you see me leaking?"

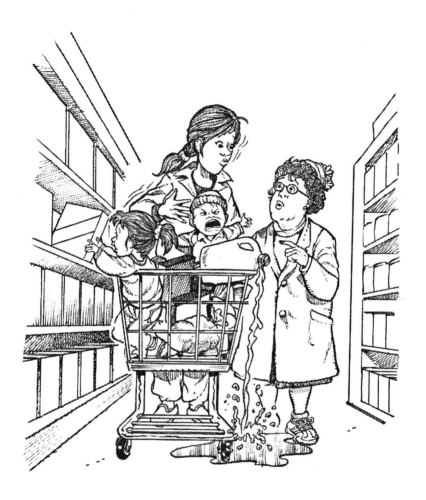

To my surprise, she was pointing at my cart, where a carton of milk had toppled over and was leaking all over the floor! My tears turned to laughter as the little old lady walked away with an exasperated expression on her face.

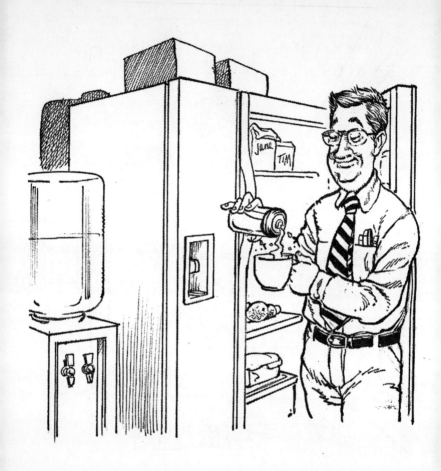

# Nonstandard Creamer

A woman at an advertising agency returned from maternity leave and sent the following e-mail:

"Whoever used the milk in the small plastic container in the refrigerator yesterday, please do NOT own up to it. I would find it forever difficult to meet your gaze across a table while having a discussion about java applets or brand identity.

"Just be aware that that milk was EXPRESSLY for my son, if you get my drift. I will label these things from now on, but if you found your coffee tasted just a little bit special, you might think of calling your mom and telling her you love her."

# Five Benefits of Mother's Milk

A young medical student took his final examination on human reproduction. After reading the first question, "Give five reasons why mother's milk is better than cow's milk for a newborn baby," he quickly wrote four answers in his exam book:

1. Mother's milk is more nutritious; it contains a better balance of fats, carbohydrates, and proteins for the newborn.
2. Mother's milk contains a mix of vitamins that aligns to a human baby's needs.
3. Mother's milk contains immunological agents that will help the newborn fight bacteria, viruses, and other infections.
4. Breastfeeding is nurturing and better developmentally for the child.

Stumped, frustrated, and running out of time, he searched his mind for a fifth reason. After pondering the question for an agonizing five minutes, he quickly scribbled a fifth reason:

5. The milk is delivered in a warm and really cute cup.

He got an A.

# Improvise

Little Edyn was only eighteen months old when her sister was born, so she was a constant companion when I was breastfeeding the baby.

One day, she decided to nurse her baby doll while I nursed her baby sister. She arranged herself next to me on the couch, carefully studying how I cradled the baby in my arm so she could do likewise. When Edyn lifted her own shirt and surveyed the lack of, um, equipment, she improvised: She stuck her elbow into the doll's mouth!

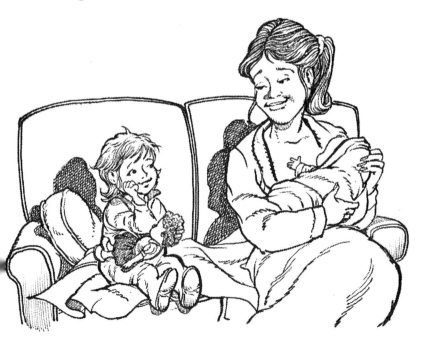

# The Queen's New Clothes

The relationship between a nursing toddler and her mother is unique. During those precious breastfeeding months, cuddling and frequent touching become the norm. Dare I say Mom becomes numbed in the chest area after awhile?

My darling Grace and I once spent a joyous afternoon grocery shopping. Oh, my timing was superb that day! We'd left home right after a nap, a quick pick-me-up cuddle, and a snack. No store displays got toppled by Grace-ful hands; she remained in a beatific mood. Beaming grandmothers made "oh, what a beautiful baby" comments. I'd managed to find everything on my shopping list, and even remembered my coupons! I was truly Supermom.

Glancing at the store clock, I realized we needed to hurry to beat the after-work crowd. As we joined the checkout line, I barely noticed the many people admiring Grace, smiling and nudging their companions to look at my precious child. Instead, I absentmindedly smiled back at them, stood just a little bit taller, and nodded graciously. This must be what it's like to be a queen, I mused to myself. The only unpleasantness was the sudden

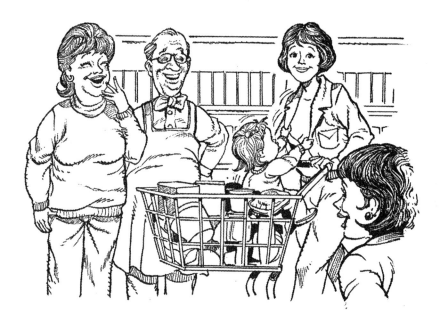

cold draft blowing in from outside. I reminded myself to pack a light jacket for Grace from now on so she wouldn't catch a chill.

When it was finally my turn to load my purchases onto the belt, I discovered it was I, not my precious child, who had been the subject of so much attention. While we were in line, Grace had gently opened all the buttons on my blouse and I was exposed to the waist.

My reverie ended. Mortified, I quickly rebuttoned my blouse as the young bagboy gave me a toothy grin and eagerly asked if I needed help with my groceries. Thanking him, I declined and slunk home to rejoin my regular peasant existence.

# 101 Uses for Breast Milk

When a friend and I first had our babies, we became interested in all the potential uses for breast milk. She used her milk to clear up her baby's acne; I used my milk to heal some fingernail scratches on my daughter's face. Our list grew and we became more inventive, even competitive. When my husband had bad road rash from a bike accident, out came my breasts. When her nephew had pinkeye, in went a squirt.

One day she asked me how I liked her homemade soap. "Very nice. My hands feel really soft," I told her. "Is it goat's milk?"

"With an added magic ingredient," she hinted.

I was beaten.

The next time we were together was at a lecture. We sat in the very back, not wanting our babies to disturb the mostly male crowd. As expected, my daughter soon began to fuss, wanting to nurse. She began to do the latch-on-latch-off routine as she kept track of the action around her. I did my best to keep up with her, but the last time she pulled off, I was too slow with the breast pad. I gave the man two rows up a healthy shot of breast milk, right on his bald crown. I was mortified and watched in horror as he reached up, rubbed his damp head, then looked up at the ceiling for a leak.

I heard my friend inhale sharply. "Wow," she whispered. "I can't believe you did that. I knew you were competitive, but I never thought you would try to cure baldness."

# Sucked the Life Out of Them

My daughter is nearly six years old, but considering the things that come from her mouth, she seems like a full-grown woman—a thirty-year-old, at the very least.

I breastfed for all the right reasons and hardly regret that my once-perky A-cups now almost kiss my stretch mark–covered stomach. Most days, I wear these sagging things like a badge.

Nevertheless, my "thirty-year-old" often makes me question this pride. A year ago, when I was still in the habit of bathing with my daughter, I sat with her in tepid bath water, eating crackers and sipping peppermint tea. We faced one another and chatted as two grown women might, until she discovered something and went stone quiet.

After she'd sorted through her thoughts, she said, "Mommy, Mommy, your breasts and bellybutton make a face...they make a face, Mommy...and the eyes are looking *down*!" She took her short index finger and shoved it down through the water to the bottom of the bathtub to punctuate her point.

We were quiet for an entire minute before I let loose my laughter and leaned against the tub in good pain. She mimicked me, and we turned red with giggles. When we finally composed ourselves, I kindly told her that *she* was responsible for my lazy breasts and that if she hadn't sucked the life from them, she'd be looking right into their "eyes." She seemed satisfied with that explanation and was probably quite proud of her jaw strength, but it wasn't until recently that I was sure I had borne a comedian.

One Saturday morning, I awoke to my daughter's serious face, her eyebrows just about meeting from worry. As usual, she was preparing to hit me with some profound revelation. She said, "Mommy, please look at your chest." I lifted my weary head and saw that both of my tiny, wrinkled, well-worked breasts had climbed out of the tank top I was so sure I'd put them in the night before.

"Put those things away," she said. "Just because I sucked the life out of them doesn't mean the whole world needs to know they're dead!"

# Mystery Bag

I wanted to be discreet about using a breast pump when I trained in my replacement as city accountant, so I left the bag in a seldom-used corner of a lobby, thinking it would go unnoticed. I couldn't have been more wrong!

Within a couple of hours, my supervisor called my office and asked if the black bag upstairs contained my breast pump.

"Yes," I replied. "Is something wrong?"

"Well..."

She went on to tell me the mayor's secretary had seen it and, not knowing whom the bag belonged to or how it got there, called the police, suspecting it to be a bomb. Two officers came and were afraid to touch the bag, so they called a special unit with an explosives-sniffing dog to the scene. Just as the dog team arrived, she and I confirmed that the bag held my breast pump, and she called off the police investigation.

But my embarrassment didn't end there. A local reporter just happened to be interviewing the city manager when he heard all the commotion. He wrote an article in the local paper entitled "Mystery bag pumps fear into City Hall." I pleaded with him not to write it, but he insisted it was a humorous story. At least he honored my request to remain anonymous!

# Speaking of the Milky Way

When my first child, Brice, was born, I immediately began referring to nursing and my "equipment" as *milky*. I had a friend whose toddler yelled *booby* when he wanted to nurse, and I wanted to avoid that embarrassment. I was not sure if Brice would nurse long enough to talk, but I figured if he did, *milky* was a nice, subtle word he could use in public.

Fast-forward fifteen months.

"Now boarding all passengers flying with young children," said the airline agent over the loudspeaker.

"That's us!" I said to my husband and Brice as we prepared to board our plane from New York to the Bahamas for vacation. We gathered up the stroller and carry-on luggage and started walking to the head of the line when suddenly Brice had a different idea about what he wanted to do. He began making the face that said he wanted to nurse.

"We'll have milky in a minute, honey," I said. Quite used to nursing on demand, Brice did not like that answer.

He began pawing at my shirt, determined to take matters into his own hands.

"I'll take him," said my husband, and we traded armfuls.

Brice was livid that he was being passed to Dad and began screaming. "Wonderful," I thought, as the other passengers began staring at us. Several even rolled their eyes, and many looked quite annoyed that there was going to be a screaming child on their flight.

Flustered and embarrassed, I told Brice, "Honey, Mommy will feed you in one minute—but we have to get on the plane first."

Brice, who could say only a few random words, began verbally articulating exactly what he wanted for the first time ever. "Balls!" he yelled. Thinking he was asking for one of his toys, I quickly searched for a ball in the diaper bag. I gave it to Brice, hoping it would quiet him.

"No!" Brice yelled, throwing the ball into the line of onlookers and reaching for my chest. "Mama balls!" Then, as if I needed further clarification as to what he wanted, he added another word to his cry: "Mama milk balls!" Realizing he was finally able to say what he wanted, his chant of "Mama mama milk balls! Mama mama milk balls!" got louder and louder until the whole line of fellow travelers also knew exactly what he wanted.

The chant continued, and laughter began rippling down the line. The annoyed looks melted and several people called out, "What a smart little guy!" and "How funny!" Their positive remarks caught Brice's attention, and his tears turned into smiles. We boarded the plane, found our seats, and finally Brice got his much desired "mama mama milk balls." He was an absolute angel the rest of the flight.

Needless to say, the word *milky* stayed behind in New York, along with any naive notion I had that a parent can control what her child says!

# In That Case...

I have a friend who's the oldest of twelve children. By the time her youngest sibling was born, she was already married. One year, the whole darn lot of them was together for a holiday meal, and the youngest, who was four at the time, sidled out of his chair in the middle of the meal and told his mother he wanted to nurse.

My friend and a couple of the older siblings had a fit. "Mom! You're still nursing him? He's too old for that. That's ridiculous!"

The mother went into a sermon about how he still enjoyed it, how she didn't want to permanently damage his little psyche, and how devastated he would be if he couldn't nurse. Finally, after much harassment from the other kids, the mother turned to her youngest and with great sorrow said, "Well, your brothers and sisters think you're too old to nurse. What do you think about that?"

The kid pondered the question for about five seconds and then asked, "Well, in that case, can I have a glass of wine?"

# The Hungry Elbow

My first child often slept many hours each night between my husband and me, and I nursed him off and on all night, rarely becoming fully awake in the process. One night I felt him moving against my body, so I pulled him close to my bare breast. But he wouldn't latch on, and he seemed to have wiggled out of his clothes. I rolled him in the loose folds of my flannel nightgown, tucked the bed sheet tightly around the edges, and pulled him even closer to keep him warm, but he still wouldn't nurse.

Finally my husband's voice penetrated my sleepy brain: "What the devil are you trying to do to me?"

I'd dragged him halfway across our king-size bed, entangled his arm in flannel and sheeting, and was desperately trying to get his elbow to nurse! Our baby was sound asleep in his crib on the far side of the room.

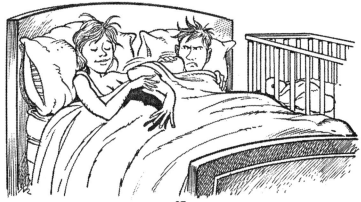

# Yeah, Baby

Five days after I started breastfeeding my first child, my milk, as they say, "came in." In fact, my breasts became so engorged that they felt and looked like two rock-hard cantaloupes. I was lucky to have a doctor's appointment that day. After wincing in sympathy, my doctor prescribed that I go straight to the nearest pharmacy, buy an electric breast pump, and put it to use.

My husband and I picked up the pump and put it together immediately, hoping for some major relief. When the pumping contraption was assembled, however, it looked like a clunky, intimidating, and potentially pain-inducing B-movie prop. By now I was even more engorged, but the fear of attaching an electrical apparatus that resembled a torture device to my sore chest prevented me from using it.

My husband tried to reassure me that it would be all right, but he failed to persuade me to "hook up." So in a moment of brilliance, my husband decided to try it out for me. He removed his T-shirt, plugged in the pump, and positioned the suction cup over his right nipple. He set the dial at the lowest setting, took

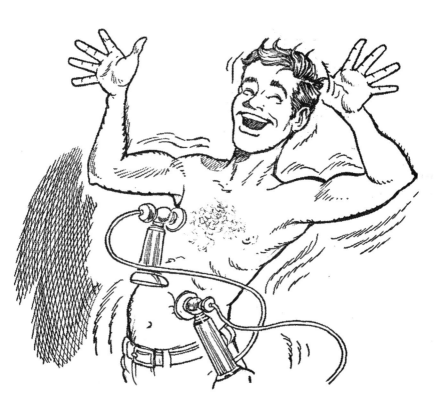

a deep breath, and hesitated momentarily before flicking on the power switch.

"Is it on?" he asked, frowning at the machine and reaching to adjust the setting. He had put on some "sympathy weight" during my pregnancy, and when he turned up the dial, the pump began sucking visible amounts of flesh into the suction cup. I started to laugh for the first time in days, and he took the opportunity to play it up for comedic effect.

With the pump on its highest setting, he began repositioning the suction cup on various parts of his upper body, eyes rolling in mock pleasure, alternating between groaning, laughing, and sarcastically saying things like, "Oh yeah, baby, that's what I'm talking about!" Through laughter I managed to snatch the pump away from him. Once I knew it wouldn't hurt, I couldn't wait to use it.

I lowered the setting and began pumping. The doctor had been right; it was just what I needed. I sat with the pump attached to me for quite a while that afternoon.

Although I don't remember talking while the pump worked its magic, if I had spoken it would have been to sigh, "Oh yeah, baby, that's what I'm talking about"— just without the sarcasm.

# From A to DD

My breasts entered the New Year's Eve party before the rest of me. No, really, they did. They were the biggest breasts I had ever owned, and they were showing the way like a couple of high beam headlights. And they were turning heads. People said "hi" to me, and then their eyes went directly to the breasts. It was a phenomenon I had never known before.

And the attention wasn't because of the way I was dressed. I had avoided overdoing the cleavage (even though I was ecstatic to actually *have* cleavage), and I was wearing a regular bra, not one of those push-'em-up-and-over ones. I had chosen a maroon silk pantsuit with a modest neckline (though the material between the breasts puckered and strained a bit).

The breasts and I spent a few hours mingling with the crowd. When I ate, they managed to keep any spilled food from landing on my lap. And dancing? Well, all of a sudden my husband decided he just loved to slow dance. But I'm not sure I would even call it dancing; it was more like breast hugging. Slow dancing seemed safer than fast dancing, though, which I would call fast bouncing. My new best friends were moving to and fro, and believe me, it was never to the beat.

Standing at the bar seemed to be a dangerous occupation for the breasts, too. When I turned, they wiped out any drinks that happened to be nearby. At last count, two martini glasses were swiped off the bar and sent crashing to the floor.

As the evening wore on, I decided to make a quick trip to the powder room. Most of my makeup still looked surprisingly good. I decided I better take a quick peek at the whole package, as long as I was there. (You know, make sure everything was tucked in and no toilet paper was stuck to my shoes.) I stepped back and turned around, first checking my pants. As I worked my way up, I gasped. There was a large, dark wet spot spreading over the front of my right breast!

I tried placing my hand over the stain, and then I noticed that my left breast was joining in on the fun. Looking around the room frantically, I spotted my sister-in-law at the end of the line. As I rushed over to her with my hands cupping the breasts, she backed away.

"I need my coat," I said. "Now! I need my coat now."

"You can't leave yet," she responded. "It's not even midnight." I noticed she slurred her words, and what I had interpreted as her backing away from me was actually her stumbling backward against the wall.

I freed the right breast from my grasp and pulled her from the line.

"My breasts are leaking," I whispered in her ear. "Please go get my coat."

"Eeeww," she said, this time really backing away from me. I shoved her through the door and watched her weave toward the coat check.

Leaning back against the bathroom wall, I noticed all eyes were on me again. I smiled nervously and crossed my arms over the breasts, trying to look casual.

When I finally got to the car, my husband helped me aim the vents in my direction, then turned the heat on full blast, hoping it would help me dry off.

At home, I ran to the bathroom and pulled off the wet, sticky top and tossed it in the sink. Leaning over the bathtub, I pulled off my bra and peeled away the soaked nursing pads, throwing them toward the waste-basket. I wiped a warm washcloth over my swollen breasts, and then patted them down with several towels until they stopped leaking.

My newborn daughter started crying, right on time for her midnight feeding, and the sound made me smile. The breasts heard her, too.

Leaning back over the edge of the tub, I looked down at my new best friends. Taking them out had proven to be a lot of trouble, but they certainly had been fun to dress up.

# The Most Important Detail

I baby-sit three little girls two days a week and bring my four-month-old son, Gerard, along. The girls—ages three, five, and seven—are all fascinated with the baby and breastfeeding.

If, as they say, imitation is the highest form of flattery, I should be flattered! The girls and their friends pretend to breastfeed their dolls and one another, playing at being me and baby Gerard. The three-year-old still sits right beside us at every feeding asking, "Where is the milk? Where? Can I see it? Where?"

The five-year-old drew a picture for me that I have displayed on my fridge at home. She drew baby Gerard and my husband—and me, in a way I never would have dreamt possible as a flat-chested teenager: I had two large, very obvious, black half-circle breasts!

When I asked her about this detail, she said matter-of-factly that she had to draw my breasts because they are so important to baby Gerard.

How true!

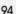

# The Great Breastfeeding Experiment

By the time our daughter was seven months old, she had been happily trained to find sustenance from my wife's breasts. She would suck with relish at long lengths, bringing perspiration to the top of her downy-haired head. My daughter never had to wait long for her feedings, as by now my wife and I were well attuned to her fussing and vocal warnings of encroaching hunger.

One afternoon, my wife had to dress quickly and depart for an evening work appointment. My daughter began fussing, and when she spied her mother putting a bra over her breasts, she must have realized a feeding was not imminent: She wailed and bawled.

I tried to comfort my daughter, but no amount of loving and snuggling would divert her attention from her growing hunger. By now, though, I was an old hand, so I gaily suggested that my wife not worry: I would retrieve a bottle of expressed milk from the fridge.

I was on my way when my wife told me she hadn't had a chance to express a new batch of breast milk. She

95

began to reach for the baby, but I told her she was late, and that I would suckle our daughter on my breast. My wife was a little incredulous, but she well knew by then that I thought nature had deprived men by not allowing us to have babies or feed them.

I placed the howling baby on the bed for a minute and took off my shirt. I told my wife that our daughter would probably be placated just by the sucking ritual, because it hadn't been long since she was last fed.

The room fell quiet as we three held a collective breath. My baby looked eagerly at my nipple. My wife looked curious and maybe a little fearful of being replaced. I felt slightly guilty that I might be committing a crime against nature as well as deceiving my unsuspecting daughter.

After a few seconds, the silence was broken. My wife laughed at my daughter's expression. I yelped in disbelief at the unexpected force of my daughter's gums clamping on my tender nipple. My daughter angrily howled and shot me a look of betrayal the likes of which I had never seen before.

My wife unhooked her bra and came to the rescue. Our daughter fell quiet amid contented sighs (punctuated every so often with glowers and growls directed at me). She soon fell asleep, my wife finished dressing, and I felt cheated as I tended to my sore nipple.

The great breastfeeding experiment was never repeated. My triumphant wife was late to her appointment, but her humming as she left told me she didn't care. Twenty-five years later, my daughter is just beginning to trust me again.

# Squirts

One day, I went to my daughter's downtown daycare on my lunch break to nurse her. A lot of moms did the same, and there were comfortable chairs and a couch for us to sit on while nursing.

The lunch hour started like any other, and the usual moms were there. I sat down on the couch and placed my baby, Draven, in the cradle position. We decided she was going to nurse from my right breast. To the left of us was another mother-daughter duo, the baby nursing from her mother's left breast.

Draven was having a difficult time latching on, and I was not letting down. I went to manually express some milk, as Draven was squirming a lot. But at that point my milk let down and, to my horror, I saw a stream of milk arc, seemingly in slow motion, right into the other baby's eye!

The mother had been looking the other way, so she didn't see her daughter get a shot of breast milk. The baby started coughing, and I could tell she was in shock. I just sat there, frozen. Finally, the mother saw the milk on her baby's face and looked at me, confused.

I don't know why, but the words that flew out of my mouth were "It wasn't me!" After a moment, I bowed my head in guilt and confessed. The other mother laughed it off and commented on the close quarters we were in. I began to feel a little relief and ventured to the group that this kind of thing must happen often. Everybody shook their heads no.

The next day as I was dropping off Draven, I saw my victim and her father. I didn't think much of the events of the previous day until the baby's father greeted me: "Good morning, squirts!"

I haven't been able to escape the nickname since.

# Credits

● ● ● ● ● ● ● ● ● ● ● ● ● ● ● ● ● ● ● ● ● ● ● ● ● ● ● ●

"101 Uses for Breast Milk" © 2007 by Diane Selkirk. Used by permission of the author.

"All Pads Are Not Created Equal" © 2007 by Mimi Greenwood Knight. Used by permission of the author.

"An Areola Never Forgets" by "princesshdrider," reprinted from StorkNet.com.

"The Buzz and the Boss" © 2007 by Alisa Gordaneer. Used by permission of the author.

"Conference Call" reprinted from www.breastfeeding.com. Copyright © 2007. Used with permission of Breastfeeding.com, Inc.

"Diagnosis" © 2007 by Ashley Beasley. Used by permission of the author.

"The Evil Twin Goes Shopping" © 2007. Used by permission of iParenting Media.

"Excuse Me, Dear..." by RoxAnne Lane Christley, reprinted from www.breastfeeding.com. Copyright © 2007. Used with permission of Breastfeeding.com, Inc.

"Five Benefits of Mother's Milk" reprinted from www.breastfeeding.com. Copyright © 2007. Used with permission of Breastfeeding.com, Inc.

"Fix-It Man" by Anonymous, reprinted from www.breastfeeding.com. Copyright © 2007. Used with permission of Breastfeeding.com, Inc.

"From A to DD" © 2007 by Tricia L. McDonald. Used by permission of the author.

"Get the Pacifier" © 2007 by Deanna M. Credle. Used by permission of the author.

"Got Cream?" by Janice Lynds, reprinted from www.breastfeeding.com. Copyright © 2007. Used with permission of Breastfeeding.com, Inc.

"Grace" by Deborah S. Hucaby Hill, reprinted from www.breastfeeding.com. Copyright © 2007. Used with permission of Breastfeeding.com, Inc.

"The Great Breastfeeding Experiment" © 2007 by Andy Plotkin. Used by permission of the author.

"Have Nipple, Will Nurse" by "mom2jazzygirl," reprinted from StorkNet.com.

"The Head Nipple Inspector" © 2007 by Patricia Parkinson. Used by permission of the author.

"How to Feed Quintuplets" reprinted from www.breastfeeding.com. Copyright © 2007. Used with permission of Breastfeeding.com, Inc.

"The Hungry Elbow" © 2007. Used by permission of iParenting Media.

"Improvise " © 2007 by S. L. "Sparki" Hansen. Used by permission of the author.

"In That Case..." by "Razz," reprinted from TheNakedOvary.com.

"Keeping Count" by Gail Vold, reprinted from www.breastfeeding.com. Copyright © 2007. Used with permission of Breastfeeding.com, Inc.